# HEALTHY EATING HACKS FOR BUSY INDIVIDUALS

## Your Roadmap to Reclaiming Control of Your Diet and Revitalizing Your Health

## Joyce M. Baker

# TABLE OF CONTENTS

# INTRODUCTION

## Unlocking the Secrets to Nourishing Your Busy Life

In the hustle and bustle of modern life, maintaining a healthy diet often feels like an insurmountable challenge. As busy individuals juggle work, family, and personal commitments, the quest for nutritious meals can easily take a backseat to convenience and time constraints. The result? A reliance on fast food, processed snacks, and microwave dinners that leave us feeling drained, sluggish, and far from our best selves.

But what if I told you that eating healthy doesn't have to be a time-consuming chore? What if I revealed a treasure trove of simple, practical strategies that can revolutionize the way you approach nutrition, even in the midst of your busiest days? Welcome to "Healthy Eating

Hacks for Busy Individuals" – your roadmap to reclaiming control of your diet and revitalizing your health, one delicious bite at a time.

In this book, we'll embark on a transformative journey together, exploring innovative hacks, savvy shortcuts, and mouthwatering recipes designed specifically for those with jam-packed schedules and limited time to spare. From mastering the art of meal prep to uncovering the hidden gems of on-the-go nutrition, each chapter is packed with actionable advice and insider tips to help you thrive in the fast-paced whirlwind of modern life.

But this book is more than just a collection of quick-fix solutions; it's a manifesto for change, a rallying cry for a healthier, happier future. It's about empowering you – the busy professional, the harried parent, the on-the-go student – to take charge of your dietary destiny and forge a path to wellness that fits seamlessly into your hectic lifestyle.

So, if you're ready to bid farewell to the drive-thru dinners and microwave meals, if you're eager to reclaim your vitality and rediscover the joy of nourishing your body, then join me on this exhilarating adventure. Together, we'll unlock the secrets to healthy eating success and embark on a journey toward a brighter, more vibrant tomorrow.

Get ready to revolutionize your approach to nutrition, one healthy hack at a time. Your journey to a healthier, happier you starts now.

# CHAPTER 1

## THE BUSY INDIVIDUAL'S DILEMMA: *Navigating Nutrition in a Fast-Paced World*

**Introduction to the challenges busy individuals face when it comes to maintaining a healthy diet.**

In today's fast-paced world, juggling multiple responsibilities has become the norm for many individuals. Whether it's balancing a demanding career, managing household chores, caring for family members, or pursuing personal goals, time often feels like a scarce commodity. Amidst this hustle and bustle, maintaining a healthy diet can easily slip down the list of priorities. However, the importance of nutrition cannot be overstated, as it directly impacts our physical health, mental well-being, and overall quality of life.

Despite the best intentions, busy individuals face a myriad of challenges when it comes to nourishing their bodies adequately. From hectic schedules to tempting convenience foods, various factors can hinder their ability to make nutritious choices consistently. In this discussion, we will explore some of the primary obstacles that busy individuals encounter on their quest for a healthy diet and examine potential strategies to overcome these challenges. By understanding these hurdles and implementing practical solutions, individuals can take proactive steps towards prioritizing their health amidst life's demands.

**Exploring common obstacles such as time constraints, convenience foods, and lack of meal preparation skills**

**Time Constraints:**

Time scarcity is perhaps the most ubiquitous challenge faced by busy individuals when it comes to maintaining a healthy diet. Balancing professional commitments, familial responsibilities, social engagements, and personal pursuits leaves little room for leisurely meal preparation and mindful eating. As a result, many individuals find themselves opting for quick-fix solutions such as fast food or pre-packaged meals, which are often laden with unhealthy ingredients and lacking in essential nutrients.

***Strategies to Overcome Time Constraints:***

- ***Prioritize meal planning:*** Dedicate a small portion of time each week to plan meals and snacks in advance. This can involve creating a weekly menu, preparing grocery lists, and even prepping ingredients ahead of time.

- ***Embrace batch cooking:*** Cook large batches of meals on weekends or during less hectic periods and portion them out for easy reheating throughout the week.

- ***Opt for time-saving cooking methods:*** Explore quick and simple cooking techniques such as stir-frying, sheet pan dinners, and one-pot meals that require minimal preparation and cleanup.

- ***Utilize convenience appliances:*** Invest in kitchen gadgets such as slow cookers, pressure cookers, and microwave steamers to streamline meal preparation and reduce cooking time.

**Convenience Foods:**

In our fast-paced society, convenience foods abound, offering quick and effortless solutions to hunger pangs and cravings. However, many of these convenience foods are highly processed, packed with preservatives, unhealthy fats, and excessive sodium, and devoid of essential nutrients. Moreover, the omnipresence of fast food restaurants, vending machines, and packaged snacks makes it all too easy for busy individuals to succumb to unhealthy temptations when pressed for time.

### *Strategies to Overcome Convenience Foods:*

- *Plan ahead for healthy alternatives:* Stock up on nutritious grab-and-go options such as fresh fruit, pre-cut vegetables, Greek yogurt, nuts, seeds, and whole-grain crackers to satisfy hunger cravings on the fly.

- *Make healthier choices when dining out:* When eating at restaurants or ordering takeout, opt for dishes that prioritize lean proteins, whole grains, and plenty of vegetables, and request modifications to reduce added fats, sugars, and sodium.

- *Limit exposure to temptation:* Minimize the presence of unhealthy convenience foods in your environment by keeping them out of sight and opting for healthier alternatives whenever possible.

## Lack of Meal Preparation Skills:

For many busy individuals, the thought of planning and preparing nutritious meals from scratch can be daunting, especially if they lack confidence in their culinary abilities. Without the necessary skills and knowledge, meal preparation may seem like a time-consuming and labor-intensive endeavor, leading individuals to rely on convenience foods or takeout options instead.

## Strategies to Overcome Lack of Meal Preparation Skills:

- ***Educate yourself:*** Take advantage of online resources, cookbooks, cooking classes, and instructional videos to learn basic cooking techniques, recipe ideas, and meal planning strategies.

- ***Start small:*** Begin by mastering a few simple recipes that require minimal ingredients and preparation steps, gradually expanding your repertoire as you gain confidence in the kitchen.

- ***Get creative with leftovers:*** Transform leftover ingredients into new meals by repurposing them in soups, salads, sandwiches, or stir-fries, reducing food waste and saving time in the process.

- ***Involve family and friends:*** Turn meal preparation into a social activity by cooking with family members, friends, or roommates, allowing you to share the workload and exchange cooking tips and ideas.

## Highlighting the importance of nutrition in overall well-being and productivity

Nutrition plays a fundamental role in shaping our physical health, mental well-being, and overall quality of life. It serves as the foundation upon which our bodies and minds thrive, providing the essential nutrients needed for optimal function and resilience. From supporting immune function and energy metabolism to promoting cognitive function and emotional stability, the impact of nutrition on our well-being cannot be overstated.

- ***Physical Health:*** A well-balanced diet rich in fruits, vegetables, whole grains, lean proteins, and healthy fats provides the necessary vitamins, minerals, antioxidants, and macronutrients to support a strong and resilient body. Adequate nutrition is essential for maintaining a healthy weight, reducing the risk of chronic diseases such as obesity, diabetes, heart disease, and certain cancers, and promoting longevity and vitality.

- ***Mental Well-being:*** The link between nutrition and mental health is increasingly recognized, with research demonstrating the profound influence of diet on mood, cognition, and emotional well-being. Nutrient-dense foods support brain health and neurotransmitter function, helping to regulate mood, alleviate stress, and enhance cognitive performance. Conversely, poor dietary choices characterized by excessive consumption of processed foods, sugar, and unhealthy fats have been associated with an increased risk of depression, anxiety, and cognitive decline.

- ***Energy and Productivity:*** Nutrition plays a crucial role in fueling our bodies and sustaining optimal energy levels throughout the day. By providing a steady supply of nutrients and calories, a balanced diet helps regulate blood sugar levels, stabilize energy levels, and prevent energy crashes and fatigue. Moreover, certain nutrients such as B vitamins, iron, and omega-3 fatty acids play key roles in energy metabolism, cognitive function, and focus, enhancing productivity and mental clarity.

- ***Immune Function:*** The immune system relies on a diverse array of nutrients to mount an effective defense against pathogens and maintain immune health. Adequate intake of vitamins, minerals, antioxidants, and phytonutrients supports immune function, reduces the risk of infections, and promotes faster recovery from illness. Conversely, poor nutrition compromises immune function, leaving individuals more susceptible to infections and illnesses.

- ***Long-term Health and Resilience:*** By prioritizing nutrition and adopting healthy eating habits, individuals can lay the groundwork for long-term health and resilience. A nutrient-rich diet not only reduces the risk of chronic diseases and age-related ailments but also enhances the body's ability to withstand stress, recover from illness, and maintain optimal function well into old age. Investing in nutrition today pays dividends in the form of improved quality of life, longevity, and overall well-being in the years to come.

Nutrition is a cornerstone of well-being and productivity, exerting a profound influence on every aspect of our physical, mental, and emotional health. By nourishing our bodies with a diverse array of nutrient-dense foods and adopting healthy eating habits, we can support our overall vitality, resilience, and productivity, enabling us to thrive in both our personal and professional endeavors.

**Setting the stage for practical strategies and hacks to overcome these challenges**

While the obstacles to maintaining a healthy diet for busy individuals are undeniable, they are by no means insurmountable. With determination, creativity, and a willingness to prioritize health, individuals can develop practical strategies and hacks to navigate these challenges effectively. By adopting a proactive approach and implementing actionable tactics, it is possible to overcome time constraints, resist the allure of convenience foods, and acquire essential meal preparation skills. Here are some key steps to set the stage for success:

- ***Mindset Shift:***

Cultivate a mindset that prioritizes health and recognizes the intrinsic value of nourishing your body with wholesome, nutrient-rich foods. View nutrition as an investment in your well-being and productivity, rather than a burdensome chore or inconvenience.

- ***Goal Setting:***

Set specific, achievable goals related to nutrition and wellness that align with your values and priorities. Whether it's incorporating more fruits and vegetables into your diet, reducing consumption of processed foods, or improving meal preparation skills, clearly define your objectives and establish a plan of action to work towards them.

- ***Time Management:***

Identify pockets of time in your schedule where you can dedicate attention to meal planning, grocery shopping, and meal preparation. Utilize time-saving strategies such as batch cooking, meal prepping, and utilizing convenience appliances to streamline the cooking process and maximize efficiency.

- ***Education and Skill Development:***
Invest time in educating yourself about nutrition, cooking techniques, and healthy eating habits. Take advantage of online resources, cookbooks, cooking classes, and instructional videos to expand your culinary repertoire and build confidence in the kitchen.

- ***Strategic Planning:***
Develop a strategic approach to meal planning and grocery shopping that minimizes waste, maximizes nutrient intake, and accommodates your busy lifestyle. Create weekly meal plans, prepare grocery lists, and shop with purpose to ensure that you have nutritious ingredients on hand when you need them.

- ***Smart Substitutions:***
Identify healthier alternatives to your favorite convenience foods and processed snacks, and stock your pantry and fridge accordingly. Experiment with nutritious grab-and-go options such as fresh fruits, vegetables, nuts, seeds, whole-grain crackers, and yogurt to satisfy cravings and sustain energy levels throughout the day.

- ***Flexibility and Adaptability:***
Be flexible and adaptable in your approach to nutrition, recognizing that life is unpredictable and circumstances may change. Embrace imperfection and allow yourself the grace to make adjustments as needed, rather than striving for unattainable perfection.

- ***Support Network:***
Surround yourself with a supportive network of family, friends, or colleagues who share your commitment to healthy living. Lean on them for encouragement, accountability, and practical

tips, and consider cooking together or sharing meals to enhance social connection and foster a sense of community.

By laying the groundwork with a positive mindset, clear goals, and practical strategies, you can overcome the challenges of maintaining a healthy diet in the midst of a busy lifestyle. With dedication and perseverance, you can cultivate habits that support your well-being, boost your productivity, and enhance your overall quality of life.

# CHAPTER 2

## MASTERING MEAL PREP: *The Key to Effortless Healthy Eating*

**Understanding the concept and benefits of meal prepping for busy lifestyles**

Meal prepping has emerged as a popular strategy for busy individuals seeking to maintain a healthy diet amidst hectic schedules and competing demands. The concept of meal prepping involves preparing and portioning out meals and snacks in advance, typically for a specific period, such as a week. These pre-prepared meals are then stored in the refrigerator or freezer, ready to be reheated and enjoyed at a moment's notice. While meal prepping requires some upfront time and effort, its numerous benefits make it a valuable tool for simplifying mealtime and supporting overall health and well-being.

### *Time-Saving Convenience:*

One of the primary advantages of meal prepping is its time-saving convenience. By dedicating a few hours on weekends or during less busy periods to prepare meals in advance, busy individuals can save valuable time during the week. With pre-prepped meals readily available, there's no need to spend time each day planning, shopping for ingredients, and cooking from scratch. Instead, individuals can simply grab a pre-portioned meal from the fridge or freezer and enjoy a nutritious, home-cooked meal with minimal effort.

### *Streamlined Meal Planning:*

Meal prepping simplifies the meal planning process by providing a structured framework for deciding what to eat throughout the week. By creating a meal plan and preparing meals in advance, individuals can avoid the stress and indecision that often accompanies last-minute meal preparation. Additionally, meal prepping allows for greater consistency in dietary choices, making it easier to adhere to health and nutrition goals.

### *Portion Control and Nutrition:*

Another benefit of meal prepping is its ability to promote portion control and facilitate healthier eating habits. By portioning out meals and snacks in advance, individuals can ensure that they consume appropriate serving sizes and avoid overeating. Moreover, meal prepping enables individuals to prioritize nutrient-dense ingredients and incorporate a variety of fruits, vegetables, lean proteins, and whole grains into their meals, thereby supporting overall nutrition and well-being.

### *Cost Savings:*

Meal prepping can also lead to significant cost savings over time. By purchasing ingredients in bulk, taking advantage of sales and discounts, and minimizing food waste through careful planning and portioning, individuals can reduce their overall grocery expenses. Additionally, by preparing meals at home rather than dining out or ordering takeout, individuals can save money on restaurant meals and convenience foods while enjoying healthier, homemade alternatives.

### *Increased Variety and Creativity:*

Contrary to popular belief, meal prepping does not have to result in monotony or repetitive eating. With a little creativity and planning, individuals can enjoy a diverse array of flavors, cuisines, and recipes throughout the week. Experimenting with different ingredients, seasonings, and cooking methods allows individuals to discover new dishes and flavors, keeping mealtime exciting and enjoyable.

### *Stress Reduction:*

Finally, meal prepping can contribute to reduced stress and greater peace of mind. By knowing that meals are already prepared and waiting, individuals can eliminate the daily pressure of deciding what to eat and scrambling to find time to cook. This sense of preparedness and organization can alleviate stress and create a sense of control over one's dietary choices, ultimately contributing to overall well-being.

Meal prepping is a valuable strategy for busy individuals seeking to prioritize health and nutrition in the midst of hectic lifestyles. By investing time and effort upfront to prepare meals in advance, individuals can enjoy the time-saving convenience, streamlined meal planning, portion control, cost savings, increased variety, and stress reduction that meal prepping offers. With careful planning and a commitment to consistency, meal prepping can empower individuals to make healthier choices, save time and money, and support their overall health and well-being.

**Step-by-step guide to effective meal planning and preparation, including batch cooking and storage tips**

## *Assess Your Needs and Preferences:*

- Begin by assessing your dietary needs, preferences, and goals. Consider factors such as dietary restrictions, food allergies, cultural preferences, and personal taste preferences.
- Determine how many meals and snacks you need to prepare for the week, taking into account your schedule, lifestyle, and anticipated time constraints.

## *Create a Weekly Meal Plan:*

- Design a weekly meal plan that incorporates a balance of macronutrients (carbohydrates, proteins, fats), as well as a variety of fruits, vegetables, whole grains, and lean proteins.
- Utilize recipes, cookbooks, online resources, and meal planning apps to generate ideas and inspiration for meals and snacks.
- Consider incorporating theme nights (e.g., Meatless Mondays, Taco Tuesdays) to

streamline meal planning and add variety to your menu.

## *Make a Detailed Grocery List:*

- Based on your meal plan, create a comprehensive grocery list that includes all the ingredients you'll need for the week's meals and snacks.
- Organize your list by food categories (e.g., produce, dairy, proteins) to streamline your shopping experience and minimize time spent in the grocery store.
- Check your pantry, fridge, and freezer for any items you already have on hand to avoid duplicate purchases and reduce food waste.

## Set Aside Time for Meal Preparation:

- Designate a specific time each week for meal preparation, such as a weekend morning or evening when you have a few hours to spare.

- Create a conducive environment for meal prep by clearing and organizing your kitchen workspace, gathering necessary cooking utensils and equipment, and putting on some music or a podcast to make the process enjoyable.

***Batch Cooking and Preparation:***
- Choose recipes that lend themselves well to batch cooking, such as soups, stews, casseroles, and one-pot meals.
- Prepare large batches of key components such as grains, proteins, and vegetables that can be used in multiple dishes throughout the week.
- Use time-saving cooking methods such as slow cookers, pressure cookers, and sheet pan cooking to streamline the cooking process and maximize efficiency.

***Portion Out Meals and Snacks:***
- Once your meals are cooked and prepared, portion them out into individual

containers or serving sizes to facilitate easy storage and reheating.
- Label containers with the name of the dish and the date it was prepared to ensure freshness and prevent confusion.
- Consider investing in reusable, microwave-safe containers with compartments for storing complete meals or snacks.

### *Proper Storage and Refrigeration:*
- Store prepped meals and snacks in airtight containers or resealable bags to maintain freshness and prevent contamination.
- Refrigerate perishable items promptly to prevent spoilage and foodborne illness.
- Utilize clear storage containers or labels to easily identify contents and expiration dates.

### *Freezing for Future Use:*
- For meals that won't be consumed within a few days, consider freezing them for future use.

- Use freezer-safe containers or resealable bags to store frozen meals, and label them with the name of the dish and the date it was prepared.
- When reheating frozen meals, allow them to thaw in the refrigerator overnight before reheating in the microwave or oven.

### *Rotate and Enjoy:*

- Incorporate variety into your meal plan by rotating different dishes and recipes throughout the week.
- Enjoy the convenience of having pre-prepared meals and snacks readily available, and savor the satisfaction of nourishing your body with homemade, nutritious food.

By following this step-by-step guide to effective meal planning and preparation, including batch cooking and storage tips, you can streamline your cooking process, save time and money, and support your health and well-being amidst a busy lifestyle. With practice and consistency, meal planning and preparation can become a rewarding and sustainable habit that empowers you to make healthier choices and enjoy delicious, homemade meals every day.

**Quick and easy meal prep recipes that can be customized to individual preferences and dietary needs**

***Quinoa Salad Bowls:***
- Cook a batch of quinoa according to package instructions and allow it to cool.
- In individual containers, layer cooked quinoa with a variety of toppings such as mixed greens, cherry tomatoes, cucumber slices, avocado chunks, shredded carrots, and roasted chickpeas or grilled chicken.
- Customize with your favorite dressing or sauce, such as balsamic vinaigrette, tahini dressing, or salsa.

### *Stir-Fry Meal Prep:*

- Prepare a large batch of your favorite stir-fry vegetables, such as bell peppers, broccoli, snap peas, carrots, and mushrooms, sautéed with garlic and ginger in a wok or skillet.
- Add protein of choice, such as tofu, chicken, shrimp, or tempeh, cooked until browned and cooked through.
- Serve with cooked brown rice, quinoa, or cauliflower rice, and portion into individual containers for easy reheating.

### *Mason Jar Salads:*

- Layer mason jars with your favorite salad ingredients, starting with dressing at the bottom and ending with leafy greens on top to prevent wilting.
- Customize with a variety of vegetables, proteins (such as grilled chicken, hard-boiled eggs, or chickpeas), grains (such as quinoa or farro), and toppings (such as nuts, seeds, and cheese).

- When ready to eat, simply shake the jar to distribute the dressing and enjoy a fresh and flavorful salad on the go.

### Veggie Egg Muffins:

- Preheat the oven to 350°F (175°C) and grease a muffin tin.
- In a large bowl, whisk together eggs and milk (or non-dairy milk) until well combined. Season with salt, pepper, and any desired herbs or spices.
- Stir in chopped vegetables such as bell peppers, spinach, onions, tomatoes, and mushrooms, as well as cooked meat or meat alternatives if desired.
- Pour the egg mixture into the prepared muffin tin, filling each cup about three-quarters full.
- Bake for 20-25 minutes or until the egg muffins are set and golden brown on top. Allow to cool before removing from the muffin tin and storing in the refrigerator.

### Buddha Bowls:

- Start with a base of cooked grains such as brown rice, quinoa, or couscous.
- Add a variety of roasted or raw vegetables, such as sweet potatoes, Brussels sprouts, cauliflower, kale, and beets.
- Include a source of protein such as grilled tofu, chickpeas, lentils, or shredded chicken.
- Drizzle with your favorite sauce or dressing, such as tahini sauce, peanut sauce, or avocado dressing, and sprinkle with toppings such as sesame seeds, chopped nuts, or fresh herbs.

### *Overnight Oats:*

- In individual jars or containers, combine rolled oats with your choice of milk (dairy or non-dairy), yogurt, or kefir.
- Add flavorings and mix-ins such as chia seeds, flaxseed meal, nut butter, honey, maple syrup, vanilla extract, cinnamon, and fresh or dried fruit.

- Stir well to combine, cover, and refrigerate overnight.
- In the morning, grab a jar of overnight oats from the fridge and enjoy a delicious and nutritious breakfast on the go.

These quick and easy meal prep recipes offer versatility and flexibility, allowing you to customize them to suit your individual preferences and dietary needs. Whether you're following a specific eating plan, accommodating food allergies or intolerances, or simply craving variety, these customizable recipes make meal prep a breeze while ensuring that you have delicious and nourishing meals ready to enjoy throughout the week.

**Time-saving hacks for grocery shopping, ingredient organization, and maximizing freshness**

**Efficient Grocery Shopping:**
- *Plan Ahead:* Create a weekly meal plan and corresponding grocery list based on

the recipes you intend to make. This helps streamline your shopping trip and ensures you have all the ingredients you need.

- ***Online Shopping:*** Consider utilizing online grocery shopping and delivery services, which can save time by allowing you to shop from the comfort of your home and have groceries delivered directly to your doorstep.

- ***Shop Off-Peak Hours:*** Avoid crowds and long checkout lines by shopping during off-peak hours, such as early mornings or late evenings.

- ***Use Grocery Apps:*** Take advantage of grocery store apps that offer digital coupons, weekly sales flyers, and shopping lists to help you find deals and stay organized.

## Ingredient Organization:

- ***Store Similar Items Together:*** Group similar ingredients together in your pantry, refrigerator, or freezer to make it easier to find what you need when meal prepping or cooking.

- ***Label Containers:*** Use clear, labeled containers to store pantry staples such as grains, legumes, nuts, and dried fruits. Labeling containers helps prevent confusion and ensures ingredients stay fresh.

- ***Prep Ingredients in Advance:*** Wash, chop, and portion out ingredients such as vegetables, fruits, and meats ahead of time, so they're ready to use when you're cooking. This saves time and makes meal preparation more efficient.

**Maximizing Freshness:**
- ***First-In, First-Out (FIFO):*** Practice the FIFO method when organizing your refrigerator and pantry by rotating older

items to the front and placing newer items in the back. This helps prevent food waste and ensures you use up perishable items before they expire.

- ***Proper Storage:*** Store perishable items such as fruits, vegetables, dairy, and meats in the appropriate storage containers or bags to maintain freshness and prevent spoilage. Utilize crisper drawers, airtight containers, and resealable bags to extend shelf life.

- ***Use Freshness Indicators:*** Check expiration dates, sell-by dates, and use-by dates on food packaging to ensure freshness. Additionally, use your senses of sight, smell, and touch to assess the quality of perishable items before consuming them.

- ***Freeze for Long-Term Storage:*** Preserve the freshness of perishable items by freezing them for long-term storage. Use freezer-safe containers or bags to store fruits, vegetables, meats, and prepared meals, and label them with the date they were frozen.

## Quick Shopping Hacks:

- ***Stick to Your List:*** Resist impulse purchases by sticking to your grocery list and avoiding unnecessary items that aren't part of your meal plan.

- ***Shop the Perimeter:*** Focus on shopping the perimeter of the grocery store, where fresh produce, meats, dairy, and whole foods are typically located. This helps minimize exposure to processed foods and encourages healthier choices.

- ***Utilize Self-Checkout:*** Save time at the checkout by utilizing self-checkout lanes when available. Self-checkout allows you to scan and bag your items quickly without waiting in line for a cashier.

By implementing these time-saving hacks for grocery shopping, ingredient organization, and maximizing freshness, you can streamline your meal preparation process, save time and money, and ensure that you always have fresh, nutritious ingredients on hand to support your healthy lifestyle.

# CHAPTER 3

## SMART SWAPS AND SUBSTITUTIONS: *Transforming Convenience Foods into Nutritious Options*

**Identifying common processed and convenience foods and their healthier alternatives**

- **Processed Meats:**

***Common Examples:*** Deli meats, sausages, bacon, hot dogs.

***Healthier Alternatives:*** Lean cuts of fresh poultry, fish, or grass-fed beef; plant-based protein options like tofu, tempeh, or legumes;

homemade deli-style meats without added preservatives.

- **Packaged Snack Foods:**

*Common Examples:* Potato chips, crackers, cookies, candy bars.

*Healthier Alternatives:* Air-popped popcorn, whole grain crackers, rice cakes; fresh fruits and vegetables with hummus or nut butter; homemade energy bites or granola bars made with natural sweeteners and whole ingredients.

- **Sugary Beverages:**

*Common Examples:* Soda, sweetened fruit juices, energy drinks.

*Healthier Alternatives:* Water infused with fresh fruit or herbs; herbal teas; sparkling water with a splash of fruit juice; homemade smoothies with whole fruits and vegetables.

- **Frozen Convenience Meals:**

*Common Examples:* Frozen pizzas, pre-packaged meals, microwave dinners.

*Healthier Alternatives:* Homemade frozen meals made with lean proteins, whole grains, and plenty of vegetables; frozen vegetables and fruits for quick stir-fries, soups, or smoothies; pre-cooked grains like quinoa or brown rice for easy meal assembly.

- **Pre-Packaged Sauces and Condiments:**
*Common Examples:* Bottled salad dressings, marinades, barbecue sauces.

*Healthier Alternatives:* Homemade salad dressings made with olive oil, vinegar, and fresh herbs; marinades with citrus juice, herbs, and spices; homemade barbecue sauce with natural sweeteners and low sodium options.

- **Refined Grain Products:**
*Common Examples:* White bread, white rice, pasta made from refined flour.

***Healthier Alternatives:*** Whole grain bread, brown rice, quinoa, whole wheat pasta; alternative grains like barley, farro, or bulgur for added variety and nutrition.

- **Processed Breakfast Cereals:**

***Common Examples:*** Sugary cereals with artificial flavors and colors.

***Healthier Alternatives:*** Whole grain cereals with minimal added sugar; oatmeal topped with fresh fruit, nuts, and seeds; homemade granola made with whole grains, nuts, and dried fruits.

By identifying common processed and convenience foods and choosing healthier alternatives, individuals can improve their dietary choices and support overall health and well-being. Making small changes to replace processed foods with whole, nutrient-dense options can lead to long-term improvements in health and vitality.

# Creative ingredient substitutions to boost nutritional value without sacrificing taste or convenience

1. ## *Swap White Flour for Whole Wheat Flour:*
   - Whole wheat flour adds fiber, vitamins, and minerals compared to refined white flour. Use it in recipes for baked goods such as bread, muffins, and pancakes for added nutritional benefits without compromising taste or texture.

2. ## *Substitute Greek Yogurt for Sour Cream or Mayonnaise:*
   - Greek yogurt is a nutritious alternative to sour cream or mayonnaise, offering protein, probiotics, and calcium. Use it in dips, dressings, and sauces for a creamy texture with a boost of nutrition.

### *3. Use Nutritional Yeast Instead of Cheese:*

- Nutritional yeast is a vegan-friendly substitute for cheese that adds a cheesy flavor and a dose of B vitamins, protein, and minerals. Sprinkle it on pasta, salads, popcorn, or casseroles for a savory boost.

### *4. Opt for Avocado Instead of Butter or Margarine:*

- Avocado is a heart-healthy alternative to butter or margarine, providing healthy fats, fiber, and vitamins. Mash avocado onto toast, use it as a spread in sandwiches, or incorporate it into baked goods for added moisture and nutrition.

### *5. Choose Zucchini or Cauliflower for Pasta or Rice:*

- Spiralized zucchini (zoodles) or grated cauliflower (cauliflower rice) make excellent substitutes for traditional pasta or rice, offering fewer carbohydrates and more vitamins and minerals. Use them in stir-fries, salads, or casseroles for a lighter, veggie-packed meal.

### 6. Replace Processed Sugars with Natural Sweeteners:

- Substitute refined sugars with natural sweeteners such as honey, maple syrup, or dates to reduce added sugars and increase antioxidants and nutrients. Use them in baking, cooking, or sweetening beverages for a healthier alternative.

### 7. Add Leafy Greens to Smoothies or Sauces:

- Incorporate leafy greens such as spinach, kale, or Swiss chard into smoothies or sauces for an extra dose of vitamins, minerals, and fiber. Their mild flavor blends well and adds nutrition without altering taste significantly.

### 8. *Include Flaxseed or Chia Seeds for Omega-3s and Fiber:*

- Boost the nutritional content of baked goods, oatmeal, yogurt, or smoothies by adding flaxseed meal or chia seeds. These seeds are rich in omega-3 fatty acids, fiber, and antioxidants, providing numerous health benefits without altering taste.

By incorporating these creative ingredient substitutions into your meals and snacks, you can enhance the nutritional value of your food while maintaining taste and convenience. Experiment with these alternatives to discover new flavors, textures, and health benefits in your favorite recipes.

## Quick and easy recipe modifications to make favorite dishes healthier and more nourishing

### 1. *Reduce Added Sugar:*

- Cut back on added sugars in recipes by using natural sweeteners like honey, maple syrup, or mashed bananas.
- Opt for unsweetened applesauce or Greek yogurt instead of sugar in baked goods for added moisture and sweetness.

### 2. *Increase Fiber:*

- Replace refined grains with whole grains like brown rice, quinoa, or whole wheat pasta to boost fiber content and promote satiety.
- Add beans, lentils, or chickpeas to soups, stews, salads, or casseroles for an extra dose of fiber and plant-based protein.

### 3. *Incorporate More Vegetables:*

- Sneak extra vegetables into favorite dishes by finely chopping or pureeing them and adding them to sauces, soups, or casseroles.
- Use spiralized vegetables like zucchini or carrots as a substitute for pasta in dishes like spaghetti or stir-fries.

### 4. Reduce Sodium:

- Cut down on sodium by using herbs, spices, citrus juice, or vinegar to add flavor to dishes instead of salt.
- Choose low-sodium or no-salt-added versions of canned goods like beans, tomatoes, and broth.

### 5. Swap Unhealthy Fats:

- Substitute unhealthy fats like butter or vegetable oil with healthier alternatives such as olive oil, avocado oil, or coconut oil.

- Use mashed avocado or nut butter in place of butter or mayonnaise in recipes like sandwiches, dressings, or baked goods.

### 6. *Increase Protein:*

- Boost protein content by adding lean sources of protein like chicken breast, tofu, tempeh, or eggs to meals and snacks.
- Incorporate Greek yogurt, cottage cheese, or protein powder into smoothies, dips, or baked goods for an extra protein boost.

### 7. *Add Nutrient-Rich Ingredients:*

- Enhance the nutritional value of dishes by adding nutrient-rich ingredients like nuts, seeds, dried fruits, or superfoods such as chia seeds, flaxseed, or hemp hearts.
- Sprinkle nutritional yeast over popcorn, salads, or pasta dishes for

a cheesy flavor and a dose of B vitamins.

## 8. *Control Portion Sizes:*

- Practice portion control by using smaller plates and bowls to help regulate serving sizes and prevent overeating.
- Fill half your plate with vegetables, one-quarter with lean protein, and one-quarter with whole grains to create balanced and nutritious meals.

By making these quick and easy recipe modifications, you can transform favorite dishes into healthier and more nourishing options without sacrificing taste or satisfaction. Experiment with these ideas to discover new flavors, textures, and health benefits in your everyday cooking.

## Tips for reading labels, choosing healthier options, and navigating restaurant menus

- ***Scan the Ingredient List:*** Focus on the ingredient list rather than just the nutrition facts. Choose products with fewer ingredients and avoid those with added sugars, unhealthy fats, and artificial additives.

- ***Check Serving Sizes:*** Pay attention to serving sizes listed on nutrition labels to ensure you're consuming appropriate portions. Be mindful of how many servings you're actually consuming to avoid overeating.

- ***Look for Whole Foods:*** Choose foods that are minimally processed and closest to their natural state. Whole grains, fruits, vegetables, lean proteins, and healthy fats are nutritious options that provide essential vitamins, minerals, and fiber.

- ***Watch for Added Sugars:*** Be wary of products that contain high amounts of added sugars, which can contribute to health issues like obesity, diabetes, and heart disease. Look for alternative sweeteners like honey, maple syrup, or stevia.

- ***Monitor Sodium Content:*** Keep an eye on sodium levels in packaged foods, as excessive sodium intake can lead to high blood pressure and other health problems. Opt for low-sodium or no-salt-added options whenever possible.

- ***Choose Lean Proteins:*** Select lean sources of protein such as poultry, fish, tofu, beans, and legumes. Limit intake of processed meats and high-fat cuts of meat, which can be higher in saturated fat and cholesterol.

- ***Prioritize Fiber-Rich Foods:*** Look for foods that are high in fiber, such as whole grains, fruits, vegetables, beans, and nuts. Fiber helps promote digestive health, regulate blood sugar levels, and keep you feeling full and satisfied.

- ***Be Mindful of Portion Sizes:*** Pay attention to portion sizes when dining out at restaurants. Consider sharing meals, ordering smaller portions, or asking for a to-go box to save leftovers for another meal.

- ***Look for Healthy Cooking Methods:*** Choose menu items that are grilled, baked, steamed, or roasted rather than fried or deep-fried. These cooking methods tend to be lower in added fats and calories.

- ***Customize Your Order:*** Don't be afraid to ask for substitutions or modifications to make your meal healthier. Requesting salad instead of fries, dressing on the side, or extra vegetables can help reduce calories and increase nutritional value.

By following these tips for reading labels, choosing healthier options, and navigating restaurant menus, you can make more informed decisions about your food choices and support your overall health and well-being.

# CHAPTER 4

## ON-THE-GO NUTRITION: *Fueling Your Body Anytime, Anywhere*

**Strategies for maintaining healthy eating habits while traveling, commuting, or working outside the home**

1. **Plan Ahead:**
   - ***Pack Healthy Snacks:*** Bring portable snacks such as fresh fruit, nuts, seeds, whole grain crackers, or granola bars to keep hunger at bay

and avoid reaching for unhealthy options while on the go.

- ***Pre-Pack Meals:*** Prepare meals in advance and pack them in reusable containers to bring with you. This allows you to control portion sizes and ensure that you have nutritious options readily available when hunger strikes.

## 2. Make Smart Choices When Eating Out:

- ***Research Restaurants:*** Look up restaurant menus ahead of time and choose places that offer healthier options such as salads, grilled proteins, and vegetable-based dishes.

- ***Ask for Modifications:*** Don't hesitate to ask for modifications to accommodate your dietary preferences or restrictions. Request grilled instead of fried, sauces on the side, or extra vegetables in place of starches.

### 3. Stay Hydrated:

- ***Carry a Water Bottle:*** Bring a reusable water bottle with you and aim to drink plenty of water throughout the day to stay hydrated and prevent dehydration, which can sometimes be mistaken for hunger.

- ***Limit Sugary Drinks:*** Be mindful of sugary beverages like soda, energy drinks, and sweetened coffee drinks, which can add empty calories and contribute to dehydration. Opt for water, herbal tea, or unsweetened beverages instead.

### 4. Practice Moderation:

- ***Enjoy Treats Mindfully:*** While it's okay to indulge in occasional treats or meals out, practice moderation and balance by focusing on portion control and savoring your indulgences without guilt.

- ***Balance Your Plate:*** Aim to include a balance of nutrients in your meals by incorporating lean proteins, whole grains, fruits, vegetables, and healthy fats. This helps keep you satisfied and energized throughout the day.

## 5. Listen to Your Body:

- ***Pay Attention to Hunger Cues:*** Tune in to your body's hunger and fullness signals and eat when you're hungry, stopping when you're satisfied. Avoid mindless eating or eating out of boredom or stress.

- ***Choose Nutrient-Dense Foods:*** Opt for nutrient-dense foods that provide sustained energy and keep you feeling full longer, such as lean proteins, fiber-rich fruits and vegetables, and whole grains.

6. **Stay Active:**
   - ***Incorporate Physical Activity:*** Find opportunities to stay active throughout the day, whether it's taking a walk during your lunch break, using the stairs instead of the elevator, or fitting in a workout before or after work. Physical activity can help support healthy eating habits and overall well-being.

By implementing these strategies for maintaining healthy eating habits while traveling, commuting, or working outside the home, you can make nutritious choices that support your health and well-being, even in busy or challenging situations.

## Portable snack ideas and recipes that provide sustained energy and nourishment on busy days

- *Trail Mix:* Combine nuts (such as almonds, walnuts, or cashews), seeds (such as pumpkin seeds or sunflower seeds), and dried fruits (such as raisins, dried cranberries, or apricots) for a satisfying and energy-boosting snack.

- *Homemade Energy Bars:* Mix together oats, nut butter, honey or maple syrup, and add-ins like chopped nuts, dried fruit, seeds, and dark chocolate chips. Press into a pan, chill, then cut into bars for a homemade snack that's packed with protein and fiber.

- *Greek Yogurt Parfait:* Layer Greek yogurt with fresh fruit (such as berries or sliced banana), granola, and a drizzle of honey or maple syrup for a nutritious and filling snack that's high in protein and calcium.

- ***Veggie Sticks with Hummus:*** Pack baby carrots, cucumber slices, bell pepper strips, and cherry tomatoes with a side of hummus for dipping. This combination provides a satisfying crunch, plenty of fiber, and protein from the hummus.

- ***Apple Slices with Nut Butter:*** Slice apples and spread them with your favorite nut butter (such as almond butter, peanut butter, or cashew butter) for a portable snack that combines sweetness with healthy fats and protein.

- ***Hard-Boiled Eggs:*** Prepare hard-boiled eggs ahead of time and pack them with a sprinkle of salt and pepper for a convenient and protein-rich snack that's perfect for on-the-go nourishment.

- ***Whole Grain Crackers with Cheese:*** Pair whole grain crackers with slices of cheese (such as cheddar, mozzarella, or goat cheese) for a satisfying snack that provides a balance of carbohydrates, protein, and healthy fats.

- ***Rice Cake with Avocado:*** Top rice cakes with mashed avocado and a sprinkle of sea salt for a simple yet satisfying snack that's rich in healthy fats, fiber, and essential nutrients.

- ***Cottage Cheese with Fruit:*** Combine cottage cheese with fresh fruit (such as pineapple, peaches, or berries) for a creamy and protein-packed snack that provides a balance of sweetness and satiety.

- ***Tuna Salad on Whole Grain Crackers:*** Mix canned tuna with Greek yogurt or avocado, diced celery, onion, and seasonings. Serve on top of whole grain crackers for a protein-rich snack that's easy to eat on the go.

These portable snack ideas and recipes provide sustained energy and nourishment on busy days, helping you stay fueled and focused throughout the day. Experiment with different combinations and flavors to find your favorites!

**Tips for making smart choices when dining out or ordering takeout while on the go**

- **Plan Ahead:**

*Research Menus:* Look up restaurant menus online before dining out or ordering takeout. This allows you to identify healthier options and make informed choices ahead of time.

*Check Reviews:* Read reviews or ask friends for recommendations to find restaurants that offer healthier options and accommodate dietary preferences or restrictions.

- **Look for Healthier Options:**

*Choose Grilled or Baked:* Opt for grilled, baked, or roasted dishes instead of fried options, which tend to be higher in unhealthy fats and calories.

***Load Up on Veggies:*** Look for dishes that are packed with vegetables or offer side salad options to increase your intake of fiber, vitamins, and minerals.

***Select Lean Proteins:*** Choose lean protein sources such as grilled chicken, fish, tofu, or beans to keep your meal balanced and satisfying.

***Be Mindful of Portions:*** Pay attention to portion sizes and avoid oversized meals by sharing dishes or asking for a smaller portion if available.

- **Customize Your Order:**

***Ask for Modifications:*** Don't hesitate to ask for substitutions or modifications to make your meal healthier. Requesting sauces on the side, extra vegetables instead of starches, or grilled instead of fried can help reduce calories and boost nutrition.

***Request Half Portions:*** If portion sizes are large, consider asking for a half portion or sharing a meal with a friend to avoid overeating.

***Skip the Extras:*** Avoid extras like bread baskets, appetizers, or sugary drinks that can add unnecessary calories and contribute to overeating.

- **Practice Portion Control:**

***Listen to Your Body:*** Pay attention to hunger and fullness cues and stop eating when you're satisfied, rather than finishing everything on your plate out of habit.

***Use Visual Cues:*** Estimate portion sizes by using visual cues, such as the size of your palm for protein, your fist for grains, and your thumb for fats.

***Save Half for Later:*** If you're served a large portion, consider saving half for later by asking for a to-go box before you start eating.

- **Watch Your Beverages:**

*Choose Wisely:* Opt for water, unsweetened tea, or other calorie-free beverages instead of sugary sodas, juices, or alcoholic drinks, which can add extra calories and sugar to your meal.

*Limit Alcohol Consumption:* Enjoy alcoholic beverages in moderation and be mindful of the calories they contribute to your overall intake.

By following these tips for making smart choices when dining out or ordering takeout while on the go, you can enjoy delicious meals while still prioritizing your health and well-being. Making informed decisions and practicing moderation can help you maintain a balanced and nutritious diet, even when eating away from home.

**Mindful eating practices to cultivate a healthy relationship with food and avoid mindless snacking**

**Eat with Awareness:**

- ***Pay Attention:*** Slow down and savor each bite, paying attention to the flavors, textures, and sensations of the food you're eating. Avoid distractions like television, phones, or computers while eating.

- ***Tune into Hunger Cues:*** Listen to your body's hunger and fullness signals, eating when you're hungry and stopping when you're satisfied. Avoid eating out of boredom, stress, or emotional triggers.

**Practice Portion Control:**

- ***Use Smaller Plates:*** Opt for smaller plates and bowls to help control portion sizes and prevent overeating. This can help trick your brain into feeling satisfied with smaller amounts of food.

- ***Measure Portions:*** Use measuring cups, spoons, or visual cues to portion out servings of food, especially calorie-dense or high-sugar items. This can help prevent mindless overeating.

## Choose Nutrient-Dense Foods:

- ***Prioritize Whole Foods:*** Focus on including a variety of whole, minimally processed foods in your diet such as fruits, vegetables, lean proteins, whole grains, and healthy fats. These foods are nutrient-rich and can help keep you feeling satisfied longer.

- ***Include Protein and Fiber:*** Aim to include protein and fiber-rich foods in each meal and snack, as they can help stabilize blood sugar levels, promote satiety, and prevent overeating.

## Identify True Hunger vs. Emotional Eating:

- ***Check-In with Yourself:*** Before reaching for a snack, ask yourself if you're truly hungry or if you're eating out of boredom, stress, or habit. Find alternative ways to cope with emotions such as taking a walk, practicing deep breathing, or engaging in a hobby.

- ***Mindful Snacking:*** If you're truly hungry between meals, opt for nutrient-dense snacks like fruits, vegetables, nuts, or Greek yogurt. Practice mindful eating even during snacks, savoring each bite and paying attention to hunger and fullness cues.

## Cultivate Gratitude and Appreciation:

- ***Practice Gratitude:*** Take a moment before eating to express gratitude for the food you're about to enjoy, acknowledging the effort that went into producing it and the nourishment it provides for your body.

- ***Appreciate the Experience:*** Approach eating as a sensory experience, appreciating the colors, aromas, and flavors of your food. Be mindful of the pleasure and satisfaction that comes from nourishing your body with wholesome foods.

## Be Gentle with Yourself:

- ***Practice Self-Compassion:*** Be kind to yourself and avoid guilt or judgment around food choices. Remember that balance and moderation are key, and it's okay to enjoy indulgent foods occasionally without feeling guilty.

By incorporating these mindful eating practices into your daily routine, you can cultivate a healthier relationship with food, prevent mindless snacking, and improve overall well-being. Mindful eating encourages you to be present in the moment, listen to your body's cues, and make choices that support your health and happiness.

# CHAPTER 5

## TIME-SAVING KITCHEN HACKS:
### *Making Healthy Cooking a Breeze*

**Clever kitchen hacks and shortcuts to streamline meal preparation and cooking time**

**Batch Cooking:**
- ***Cook Once, Eat Twice:*** Prepare larger quantities of staple ingredients like grains, proteins, and vegetables and use them in multiple meals throughout the week to save time and effort.

- ***Freeze in Portions:*** Divide batch-cooked meals into individual portions and freeze them for quick and easy meals on busy days. Label containers with the date and contents for easy identification.

## Prep in Advance:

- ***Chop and Prep Ingredients:*** Spend a few minutes each week washing, chopping, and prepping fruits, vegetables, and proteins. Store them in airtight containers or bags in the refrigerator for easy access when cooking.

- ***Make Meal Kits:*** Pre-portion ingredients for recipes into containers or bags and store them together in the refrigerator. This makes assembling meals quick and convenient, especially on busy weeknights.

## Use Time-Saving Appliances:

- ***Instant Pot:*** Utilize a multi-functional pressure cooker like the Instant Pot to cook meals quickly and efficiently. It can sauté, steam, pressure cook, and slow cook, reducing cooking time for many dishes.

- ***Slow Cooker:*** Set up ingredients in the morning and let them cook slowly throughout the day in a slow cooker. Return home to a delicious, ready-to-eat meal with minimal effort.

- ***Air Fryer:*** Use an air fryer to quickly and evenly cook foods with less oil, resulting in crispy and flavorful dishes in a fraction of the time of traditional frying methods.

## Hack Your Tools:

- ***Use Kitchen Shears:*** Save time by using kitchen shears to quickly chop herbs, trim vegetables, or cut meat directly in the pan.
- ***Grate Butter:*** Grate cold butter using a cheese grater for faster melting and easier incorporation into baked goods or sauces.

- ***Microwave Citrus:*** Microwave citrus fruits for a few seconds before juicing to make them easier to juice and extract more juice with less effort.

## Minimize Cleanup:

- ***Line Baking Sheets:*** Line baking sheets with parchment paper or aluminum foil before roasting or baking to make cleanup a breeze.

- ***One-Pot Meals:*** Choose recipes that require only one pot or pan for cooking to minimize dishes and cleanup time.

- ***Use Slow Cooker Liners:*** Line your slow cooker with a disposable liner before adding ingredients to make cleanup quick and easy.

## Repurpose Leftovers:

- ***Reinvent Meals:*** Transform leftovers into new dishes by incorporating them into salads, wraps, stir-fries, or casseroles. Get creative with flavor combinations to keep meals exciting.

- ***Freeze Extras:*** If you have leftover portions of meals, freeze them in individual containers for future quick and convenient meals.

By incorporating these clever kitchen hacks and shortcuts into your meal preparation routine, you can streamline cooking time, minimize cleanup, and make the most of your time in the kitchen, allowing you to enjoy delicious homemade meals with less stress and effort.

**Kitchen gadgets and tools that can simplify cooking tasks and save valuable time**

**Food Processor:**

*Ideal for:* Chopping, slicing, shredding, pureeing, and mixing ingredients quickly and efficiently.

*Uses:* Make homemade salsa, hummus, nut butter, dough, and more with minimal effort.

## Immersion Blender:

***Ideal for:*** Blending soups, sauces, smoothies, and dips directly in the pot or container.

*Uses:* Easily puree soups, whip up smoothies, and blend sauces without transferring to a separate blender.

## Stand Mixer:

***Ideal for:*** Mixing, kneading, and whipping ingredients for baking and cooking.

*Uses:* Make bread dough, cake batter, whipped cream, and meringue effortlessly with various attachments.

## Instant Read Thermometer:

***Ideal for:*** Quickly and accurately measuring the internal temperature of food to ensure proper cooking.

***Uses:*** Check the doneness of meat, poultry, fish, and baked goods for safe consumption.

## Mandoline Slicer:

***Ideal for:*** Slicing fruits and vegetables evenly and quickly.

***Uses:*** Create uniform slices for salads, gratins, garnishes, and more with adjustable thickness settings.

## Electric Pressure Cooker (e.g., Instant Pot):

***Ideal for:*** Cooking meals quickly under pressure with minimal supervision.

***Uses:*** Prepare soups, stews, rice, beans, and even desserts in a fraction of the time compared to traditional cooking methods.

## Air Fryer:

*Ideal for:* Frying, roasting, baking, and grilling foods with hot air circulation and minimal oil.

*Uses:* Enjoy crispy and healthier versions of fried foods like French fries, chicken wings, and vegetables without the mess of deep frying.

## Herb Stripper:

*Ideal for:* Quickly and efficiently removing leaves from herbs like thyme, rosemary, and kale.

*Uses:* Save time and effort when prepping herbs for cooking or garnishing dishes.

## Garlic Press:

*Ideal for:* Crushing garlic cloves quickly and easily without the need for chopping.

*Uses:* Add fresh garlic flavor to dishes like pasta sauces, marinades, and stir-fries with minimal cleanup.

**Silicone Baking Mats:**

*Ideal for:* Lining baking sheets to prevent sticking and promote even baking.

*Uses:* Bake cookies, pastries, and other baked goods without the need for parchment paper or greasing pans.

By investing in these kitchen gadgets and tools, you can simplify cooking tasks, save time, and enhance your efficiency in the kitchen. Whether you're chopping, mixing, blending, or cooking, these tools can help you achieve professional-quality results with less effort and more convenience.

**Tips for efficient meal assembly, multitasking, and maximizing kitchen space and resources**

**Plan Ahead:**

- *Create a Weekly Meal Plan:* Plan your meals for the week in advance to streamline grocery shopping and meal preparation. Include recipes that use similar ingredients to minimize waste and maximize efficiency.

- ***Prep Ingredients in Advance:*** Wash, chop, and portion out ingredients ahead of time to save time during meal assembly. Store prepped ingredients in airtight containers or bags in the refrigerator for easy access.

## Multitask Wisely:

- ***Use Multiple Burners:*** Cook multiple components of a meal simultaneously by utilizing different burners on the stovetop. For example, boil pasta on one burner while sautéing vegetables on another.

- ***Oven Efficiency:*** Make use of the oven's multiple racks by cooking different dishes at the same time, adjusting cooking times and temperatures as needed.

- ***Time Management:*** Plan your cooking tasks strategically to maximize efficiency. Start with longer-cooking items first, then move on to quicker-cooking components while the others continue to cook.

## Organize Your Kitchen Space:

- ***Declutter Countertops:*** Keep countertops clear of clutter to create more workspace for meal assembly. Store frequently used utensils, tools, and appliances within easy reach for quick access.

- ***Utilize Vertical Storage:*** Maximize cabinet and pantry space by using vertical storage solutions such as stackable shelves, hanging racks, or door-mounted organizers.

- ***Label and Organize:*** Label containers, jars, and storage bins to easily identify ingredients and reduce time spent searching for items. Organize your pantry and refrigerator by food category for efficient meal planning and assembly.

## Make Use of Kitchen Tools and Appliances:

- ***Invest in Time-Saving Tools:*** Use kitchen gadgets and appliances such as food processors, immersion blenders, and slow cookers to simplify meal preparation tasks like chopping, blending, and cooking.

- ***Optimize Use of Cookware:*** Choose versatile cookware and tools that can perform multiple functions. For example, a large skillet can be used for sautéing, frying, and even baking.

## Minimize Cleanup:

- ***Clean as You Go:*** Wash utensils, cutting boards, and other tools as you cook to minimize cleanup time afterward. Keep a sink or basin filled with hot, soapy water for soaking dishes while you cook.

- ***Use Disposable Liners:*** Line baking sheets, pans, and slow cookers with parchment paper, aluminum foil, or slow cooker liners to make cleanup easier and reduce scrubbing.

By implementing these tips for efficient meal assembly, multitasking, and maximizing kitchen space and resources, you can streamline your cooking process, save time, and enjoy stress-free meal preparation in your kitchen.

**Organization strategies to maintain a well-stocked pantry, fridge, and freezer for easy meal planning and preparation**

**Inventory Management:**

- ***Regularly Take Stock:*** Set aside time each week to review the contents of your pantry, fridge, and freezer. Take note of items that need replenishing or are nearing expiration.

- ***Keep a List:*** Maintain a running grocery list to jot down items as you run out of them. Organize the list by category (e.g., grains, canned goods, produce) to make shopping more efficient.

## Categorization and Labeling:

- ***Group Similar Items:*** Arrange pantry shelves, fridge compartments, and freezer bins by category (e.g., grains, beans, sauces, dairy) to streamline meal planning and preparation.

- ***Label Containers:*** Label jars, bins, and containers with the contents and expiration dates to easily identify items and prevent food waste.

## Maximize Visibility and Accessibility:

- ***Front and Center:*** Place frequently used items at eye level or within easy reach for quick access. Reserve lower shelves for heavier items and upper shelves for lighter, less frequently used items.

- ***Clear Containers:*** Store ingredients like grains, nuts, and dried fruits in clear, airtight containers to keep them fresh and easily visible. Use stackable containers to maximize vertical space.

**Rotation System:**

- ***First In, First Out (FIFO):*** Practice FIFO rotation to ensure older items are used first before newer ones. When restocking, place newer items behind older ones to encourage rotation and prevent items from expiring.
- ***Regular Purging:*** Regularly check expiration dates and remove expired or stale items from your pantry, fridge, and freezer. Donate non-perishable items that are still safe to eat but unlikely to be used.

**Utilize Storage Solutions:**

- ***Adjustable Shelving:*** Install adjustable shelving in your pantry to accommodate items of various sizes and heights.

Customize shelf heights to maximize vertical space and prevent wasted space.

- ***Baskets and Bins:*** Use baskets, bins, and drawer organizers to corral small items and keep them organized. Label containers for easy identification and access.

- ***Door Storage:*** Maximize door space with over-the-door organizers, hooks, or racks for storing spices, condiments, and other small items.

**Meal Prep and Batch Cooking:**
- ***Plan Ahead:*** Use your well-stocked pantry, fridge, and freezer as a foundation for meal planning. Plan meals based on ingredients you already have on hand to minimize waste and save time.

- ***Batch Cooking:*** Cook larger quantities of meals and freeze leftovers in portion-sized containers for future meals. Label containers with the date and contents for easy identification.

By implementing these organization strategies, you can maintain a well-stocked pantry, fridge, and freezer that supports easy meal planning and preparation. With a well-organized and efficiently stocked kitchen, you'll spend less time searching for ingredients and more time enjoying delicious homemade meals.

# CHAPTER 6

## MINDFUL EATING: *Savoring Every Bite and Cultivating Food Awareness*

**Exploring the concept of mindful eating and its benefits for physical and mental well-being**
Mindful eating is a practice that involves paying full attention to the experience of eating and drinking, without judgment or distraction. It involves being fully present in the moment and engaging all your senses while consuming food, from the sight and smell of the food to the taste and texture as you chew and swallow.

Here are some key aspects of mindful eating and its benefits for physical and mental well-being:

***Awareness of Hunger and Fullness:*** Mindful eating encourages tuning in to your body's hunger and fullness cues, allowing you to eat when you're hungry and stop when you're satisfied. This helps prevent overeating and promotes a more balanced approach to food consumption.

***Increased Satisfaction and Enjoyment:*** By slowing down and savoring each bite, mindful eating enhances the enjoyment and satisfaction derived from food. You become more attuned to the flavors, textures, and aromas of your meals, leading to a greater sense of fulfillment.

***Improved Digestion:*** Mindful eating involves chewing food thoroughly and paying attention to the process of digestion. This aids in proper digestion and nutrient absorption, reducing the likelihood of digestive discomfort such as bloating or indigestion.

***Enhanced Mind-Body Connection:*** Engaging in mindful eating fosters a deeper connection between your mind and body. You become more attuned to how different foods make you feel physically and emotionally, allowing you to make more conscious choices that support your overall well-being.

***Reduced Stress and Anxiety:*** Mindful eating can help reduce stress and anxiety surrounding food and eating. By cultivating a non-judgmental attitude towards food choices and eating habits, you develop a healthier relationship with food and alleviate feelings of guilt or shame.

***Prevention of Emotional Eating:*** Mindful eating encourages exploring the underlying emotions and triggers behind eating habits. By becoming more aware of emotional cues that drive eating behavior, you can develop healthier coping strategies and address emotional needs without resorting to food.

***Weight Management:*** Studies have shown that practicing mindful eating can support weight management goals by promoting healthier eating behaviors and reducing mindless eating. By eating more mindfully, individuals may naturally consume fewer calories and make more nutritious food choices.

***Cultivation of Gratitude and Appreciation:*** Mindful eating fosters a sense of gratitude and appreciation for the abundance of nourishing foods available. It encourages acknowledging the effort and resources that went into producing the food you consume, fostering a deeper sense of connection to food and its origins.

Overall, incorporating mindful eating practices into your daily life can lead to profound physical and mental benefits, including improved digestion, reduced stress, and a greater appreciation for the nourishing qualities of food. By bringing mindfulness to the act of eating, you can cultivate a healthier relationship with food and enhance your overall well-being.

## Techniques for practicing mindfulness during meals to enhance satisfaction and enjoyment

- ***Pause and Breathe:*** Before beginning your meal, take a moment to pause and take a few deep breaths. This helps to center yourself and bring your focus to the present moment.

- ***Engage Your Senses:*** Notice the appearance, colors, and textures of the food on your plate. Take in the aroma and appreciate the smells wafting from your meal. Engaging your senses fully can enhance your enjoyment of the eating experience.

- ***Chew Slowly and Thoroughly:*** Chew each bite of food slowly and thoroughly, savoring the flavors and textures. Pay attention to the sensation of chewing and the changing taste as you continue to chew.

- ***Put Down Utensils Between Bites:*** Instead of continuously eating without pause, put down your utensils between bites. This allows you to fully experience each mouthful and prevents mindless eating.

- ***Mindful Eating Meditation:*** Practice a brief mindfulness meditation before eating to cultivate a sense of presence and awareness. Focus on your breath or scan your body for any areas of tension before turning your attention to your meal.

- ***Check-In with Hunger and Fullness:*** Throughout your meal, periodically check in with your body to assess your hunger and fullness levels. Pause and ask yourself how hungry you are before taking another bite, and stop eating when you feel satisfied.

- ***Notice Thoughts and Emotions:*** Pay attention to any thoughts or emotions that arise while eating. Notice any judgments or reactions you have towards the food or your eating habits without attaching to them. Simply observe and let them pass.

- ***Practice Gratitude:*** Cultivate a sense of gratitude for the food on your plate and the nourishment it provides. Take a moment to appreciate the effort that went into preparing the meal and the abundance of food available to you.

- ***Minimize Distractions:*** Create a conducive environment for mindful eating by minimizing distractions such as television, phones, or reading materials. Focus your attention solely on the act of eating and the experience of nourishing your body.

- ***Practice Mindful Eating Rituals:*** Establish rituals around mealtime, such as saying a brief grace or expressing gratitude before eating. These rituals can help anchor you in the present moment and create a sense of intentionality around eating.

By incorporating these techniques into your meals, you can cultivate a greater sense of mindfulness, enhance satisfaction and enjoyment, and develop a healthier relationship with food. Mindful eating allows you to fully experience the nourishment and pleasure of each meal, leading to greater overall well-being.

**Strategies for overcoming emotional eating, stress-related eating, and other common barriers to mindful eating**

- ***Identify Triggers:*** Recognize the emotions, situations, or triggers that lead to emotional or stress-related eating. Common triggers include boredom, loneliness, anxiety, and stress. Keeping a food journal can help identify patterns and triggers.

- ***Practice Mindful Awareness:*** Increase your awareness of emotional and stress-related eating patterns by tuning into your thoughts, feelings, and bodily sensations. Notice when you're feeling the urge to eat in response to emotions rather than physical hunger.

- ***Develop Coping Strategies:*** Build a toolbox of alternative coping strategies to manage emotions and stress without turning to food. Strategies may include deep breathing exercises, meditation, journaling, going for a walk, or engaging in a hobby or activity you enjoy.

- ***Pause Before Eating:*** When you feel the urge to eat in response to emotions, pause and take a moment to check in with yourself. Ask yourself if you're physically hungry or if you're seeking comfort or distraction from emotions.

- ***Practice Self-Compassion:*** Be gentle and compassionate with yourself when faced with emotional eating urges. Instead of judging yourself harshly, acknowledge your feelings with kindness and compassion. Remember that it's okay to experience emotions and that food is not the only way to cope.

- ***Create a Support System:*** Reach out to friends, family members, or a therapist for support when dealing with emotional or stress-related eating. Having someone to talk to can provide perspective, validation, and encouragement.

- ***Mindful Eating Techniques:*** Practice mindful eating techniques to cultivate a greater awareness of your eating habits and behaviors. Pay attention to physical hunger cues, savor the flavors and textures of your food, and eat slowly and with intention.

- ***Address Underlying Issues:*** Explore underlying issues that may contribute to emotional or stress-related eating, such as unresolved emotions, past traumas, or negative self-image. Consider seeking professional help or therapy to address these issues and develop healthier coping mechanisms.

- ***Practice Stress Management:*** Incorporate stress-reducing practices into your daily routine, such as exercise, yoga, meditation, or relaxation techniques. Managing stress effectively can reduce the likelihood of turning to food for comfort.

- ***Cultivate Mindful Awareness:*** Practice mindfulness techniques throughout the day to increase overall awareness and presence. By cultivating mindfulness in daily life, you'll be better equipped to recognize and respond to emotional eating triggers with greater awareness and self-awareness.

By implementing these strategies, you can overcome emotional eating, stress-related eating, and other common barriers to mindful eating.

With practice and patience, you can develop a healthier relationship with food and cultivate greater mindfulness around eating habits and behaviors.

**Incorporating mindfulness practices into daily routines to foster a healthier relationship with food and promote mindful food choices**

- *Morning Mindfulness:* Start your day with a mindful moment. Before getting out of bed, take a few deep breaths and set an intention for the day. Use this time to center yourself and cultivate a sense of gratitude for the nourishment your body will receive.

- *Mindful Meal Planning:* Approach meal planning with mindfulness by considering the nutritional value and variety of foods you'll incorporate into your meals. Take time to plan balanced meals that include a mix of fruits, vegetables, whole grains, lean proteins, and healthy fats.

- ***Mindful Grocery Shopping:*** Practice mindfulness while grocery shopping by being fully present and attentive to your surroundings. Take time to read food labels, choose fresh, whole foods, and select items that align with your health and nutrition goals.

- ***Cooking with Presence:*** Engage in mindful cooking by being fully present and attentive to the task at hand. Take time to chop vegetables, measure ingredients, and stir pots with awareness and intention. Use this time to appreciate the colors, textures, and aromas of the foods you're preparing.

- ***Mindful Eating Rituals:*** Establish mindful eating rituals before meals, such as saying a blessing or expressing gratitude for the food on your plate. Take a moment to pause and connect with your breath before taking the first bite.

- ***Slow Down and Savor:*** Eat slowly and mindfully, taking time to chew each bite thoroughly and savor the flavors of the food. Put down your utensils between bites and pay attention to the sensations of hunger and fullness.

- ***Tune into Hunger Cues:*** Listen to your body's hunger and fullness cues before, during, and after meals. Eat when you're physically hungry and stop when you're satisfied, rather than relying on external cues or emotions to dictate your eating habits.

- ***Mindful Snacking:*** Approach snacking with mindfulness by choosing nutrient-dense foods that nourish your body and satisfy your hunger. Pay attention to portion sizes and avoid mindless snacking out of boredom or emotional triggers.

- ***Practice Gratitude:*** Cultivate a sense of gratitude for the food on your plate and the resources that went into producing it. Take a moment to express gratitude before and after meals, acknowledging the abundance of nourishing foods available to you.

- ***Evening Reflection:*** End your day with a brief mindfulness practice to reflect on your eating experiences and choices. Take a moment to acknowledge any challenges or successes you encountered and set intentions for practicing mindfulness in the days ahead.

By incorporating these mindfulness practices into your daily routines, you can foster a healthier relationship with food, promote mindful food choices, and cultivate greater awareness and appreciation for the nourishment and pleasure that food provides. Mindful eating allows you to approach food with intention, presence, and gratitude, leading to greater overall well-being.

# CONCLUSION

In conclusion, "Healthy Eating Hacks for Busy Individuals" serves as a comprehensive roadmap for individuals seeking to reclaim control of their diet and revitalize their health in the midst of hectic schedules and demanding lifestyles. Throughout the book, readers are equipped with practical strategies, innovative tips, and mindful approaches to navigate common challenges such as time constraints, convenience foods, and lack of meal preparation skills.

By embracing the principles outlined in this guide, readers are empowered to make informed choices and implement effective solutions to overcome barriers to healthy eating. From mastering the art of meal planning and preparation to incorporating mindfulness practices into daily routines, each chapter offers actionable insights and actionable steps to foster a healthier relationship with food.

Moreover, the book emphasizes the importance of nutrition in overall well-being and productivity, highlighting the transformative impact that mindful eating can have on physical and mental health. Through mindful awareness and conscious consumption, individuals can cultivate a deeper connection to their bodies, enhance satisfaction and enjoyment of meals, and ultimately achieve long-term wellness goals.

"Healthy Eating Hacks for Busy Individuals" is more than just a guide—it's a catalyst for positive change, inspiring readers to prioritize their health and well-being one delicious bite at a time. By embracing the principles of mindful eating and implementing the practical strategies outlined in this book, readers can embark on a journey towards vibrant health, renewed energy, and a revitalized sense of vitality.

www.ingramcontent.com/pod-product-compliance
Lightning Source LLC
Chambersburg PA
CBHW070821260726
48660CB00005B/1942